Table of Contents

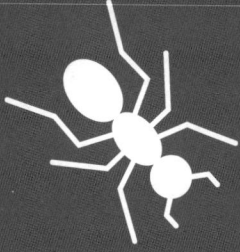

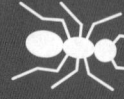

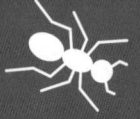

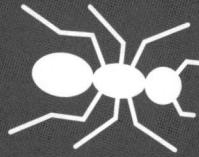

What Are ANTs?

In the early '90s, I coined the term automatic negative thoughts to describe how negativity can infest your brain.

The idea came to me after a hard day at work where I had seen 4 suicidal patients, 2 teenagers who ran away from home, and 2 couples who hated their spouses. When I got home that night, there was an ant infestation in my kitchen, where thousands of these insects were trying to take over. As I cleaned them up, the idea came to me that my patients were also infested with ANTs (automatic negative thoughts) that were driving their feelings of anxiety, depression, hopelessness, helplessness, and irritability.

My patients were infested with **ANTs (automatic negative thoughts)** that were driving their feelings of anxiety, depression, hopelessness, helplessness, and irritability.

I knew that if I could teach my patients to eliminate the ANTs, they would feel happier, less anxious, and be better able to get along with others. The next day, I brought a can of ant spray to work and started to teach my patients how to kill the ANTs. Over time, I replaced the ant spray with ant and anteater puppets, which I still use to this day. Early on I saw an 8-year-old boy who had a dog phobia and was filled with fearful thoughts about dogs. Just 3 weeks after I taught him to kill the ANTs, he told me it was an ANT ghost town in his head.

My ANT killing process is based on the work of 2 mentors: psychiatrist Aaron Beck, who pioneered a school of psychotherapy called cognitive behavior therapy (CBT), which is an effective treatment for anxiety disorders, depression, relationship problems, and even obesity; and Byron Katie, a teacher and author who developed the 5 questions we'll discuss to kill ANTs. But first, you need to understand why it's so important to eliminate the ANTs.

How ANTs Can Steal Your Happiness

How you feel is often related to the quality of your thoughts. Negative thoughts cause your brain to immediately release chemicals that affect every cell in your body, making you feel bad. The opposite is also true—positive, happy, hopeful thoughts release chemicals that make you feel good. If your thoughts are mostly negative, you will feel mostly negative; if they are mostly positive, you will feel mostly positive.

Thoughts are also automatic. They just happen.

Just because you have a thought has nothing to do with whether it is true. Thoughts lie. They lie a lot, and it is your uninvestigated or unquestioned thoughts that steal your happiness.

If you do not question or correct your erroneous thoughts, you believe them, and you act as if they are 100% true. For example, if I had the thought, My wife never listens to me, it would make me feel sad and lonely. If I never questioned the negative thought, even though it isn't true, I would act as if it were true and give myself permission to be irritable with her, making it less likely she would ever want to listen to me. Allowing yourself to believe every thought you have is the prescription for anxiety disorders, depression, relationship problems, and chronic illness. You must protect yourself from the thoughts that steal your happiness.

ANTs can link, stack, and multiply with other ANTs to attack you. For instance, the ANTs grow stronger and increase in number before bed, when you get less sleep, when your blood sugar is low, in winter, right before a woman's menstrual cycle, when you're under stress, and when you lose someone you love. This was evident during the pandemic when the spread of COVID-19 led to a rampant rise in unhealthy thinking patterns. As I said in several Facebook Live chats, in a pandemic, mental hygiene is just as important as washing your hands. We need to disinfect our thoughts.

Mental hygiene is just as important as washing your hands.
We need to disinfect our thoughts.

Look at my patient Jimmy, 39, a high-level business executive, who is featured in my book Your Brain Is Always Listening. When I first met him, he had just been released from a psychiatric hospital that morning and looked anxious and worn out. A week prior he'd told an emergency room doctor he had thought of killing himself to end the feelings of dread, panic, anxiety, and hopelessness that just wouldn't go away.

The current "episode" that brought Jimmy to the ER started 2 weeks before when he found out he had to give a presentation to one of his company's largest customers. It filled him with dread. He told me, "If I had to describe the fear, it's like you're on death row and the clock's run out. The guard opens the door and you must take the first step—that kind of fear runs through my bones."

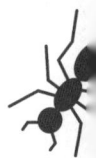

Jimmy had struggled with glossophobia (the fear of public speaking) since middle school. Through an exercise called Break the Bonds of the Past, we learned that this fear started when he was 12, the day his grandmother made him give an "impact statement" at the Los Angeles County Superior Court about why his father, one of the leaders of a violent street gang, should not get the death penalty for a double homicide. Jimmy was attacked by ANTs, including, *What if I cannot speak in court and end up killing my father?*

Even though Jimmy had repressed the memory, he had gone to great lengths throughout his life to avoid any presentations until about 6 years before when his supervisor asked him to give a brief talk at work about his role in the company. He loved his job but ruminated for days about how he would be unable to put his thoughts into words. Even after giving the presentation, the ANTs multiplied, stacked on top of one another, and attacked him, linking to many other catastrophic thoughts, such as:

> *I can't speak in public.*
> *So I'm going to lose my job.*
> *I'm going to be afraid of interviewing.*
> *So I won't be able to get a new job.*
> *I'm a loser.*
> *My wife will divorce me.*
> *I'll end up on the streets.*
> *I should kill myself*

Thankfully, Jimmy didn't act on this life-threatening ANT. By learning to kill the ANTs, Jimmy was able to feel better about himself, improve his moods, and reduce his anxiety. You can too.

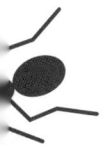

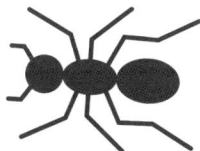

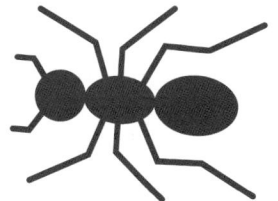

Get to Know the Most Common ANTs

Over the years, therapists have identified a number of different "species" of ANTs or types of negative thought patterns that keep your mind off balance. Here are 9 of the most common ANTs that provide the fuel for anxiety, depression, negativity, failure, relationship problems, and other emotional distress.

9 Types of ANT Species

ANT SPECIES	TYPES OF THOUGHTS	EXAMPLES
All or Nothing	Thinking that things are either all good or all bad	"Nothing ever works out for me."
Less Than	Where you compare and see yourself less than others	"I'm not smart enough."
Just the Bad	Seeing only the bad in a situation	"The world is more dangerous than ever."
Guilt Beating	Thinking in words like *should, must, ought,* or *have to*	"I should visit my parents more often."
Labeling	Attaching a negative label to yourself or someone else	"He's a jerk."
Fortune Telling	Predicting the worst possible outcome for a situation with little or no evidence for it	"I'm doomed to be unemployed for years."
Mind Reading	Believing you know what other people are thinking even though they haven't told you	"My boss doesn't like me."
If Only and I'll Be Happy When	Where you argue with the past and long for the future	"If only my parents had been rich."
Blaming	Blaming someone or something else for your problems	"It's your fault that I'm in this situation."

Learn to Kill the ANTs

Now it's time to learn how to eliminate the ANTs to be better able to cope with whatever stresses come your way. Whenever you feel sad, mad, nervous, or out of control, follow these simple steps:

1. Write down your automatic negative thoughts (ANTs). The act of writing down the ANTs helps to get the invaders out of your head.

2. Identify the ANT type(s). Use the chart to identify your ANTs.

3. Ask yourself 5 questions. These questions are life-changing. When you answer them, there are no right or wrong answers; they are just questions to open your mind to alternative possibilities. Meditate on each answer to see how they make you feel. Ask if your stressful thoughts make your life better or worse.

The 5 Questions Are:

■ QUESTION #1

Is it true? *Sometimes this first question will stop the ANT because you already know it's not true. Sometimes your answer will be "I don't know." If you don't know, then do not act like the negative thought is true. Sometimes you may think or feel that the negative thought is true, but that is why the second question is so important.*

■ QUESTION #2
Is it absolutely true with 100% certainty?

■ QUESTION #3
How do I feel when I believe this thought?

■ QUESTION #4
How would I feel if I couldn't have this thought?

■ QUESTION #5
Turn the thought around to its exact opposite, and then ask if the opposite of the thought is true or even truer than the original thought.

*Then use this turnaround as a meditation.

ANT Killing Examples

Look at the following examples to see how others have killed their ANTs.

Example #1

During the pandemic, one of my patients called in a panic because she lost her job and said:

"I'll never be able to work again."

ANT: I'll never be able to work again.

ANT Type(s): Fortune-Telling

1. Is it true? Yes.

2. Is it absolutely true with 100 percent certainty?
No, I already have part-time work lined up.

3. How do I feel when I believe this thought? Trapped, victimized, helpless.

4. How would I feel if I couldn't have the thought? Massively relieved, happy, joyful, free, like my usual self.

5. Turn the thought around to its exact opposite: I can get work again.
Any evidence that that's true? I have valuable skills that will help me get a job.

THOUGHT TO MEDITATE ON:

I have valuable skills that will help me get a job.

Example #2

From a man suffering with severe depression, one of his most toxic ANTs was:

> ## "I'm going to end up like my father who abandoned us."
>
> ANT: I'm going to end up like my father who abandoned us.
>
> ANT Type(s): Fortune-Telling

1. Is it true? No.

2. Is it absolutely true with 100 percent certainty? No, I will always be here for my chilren and wife.

3. How do I feel when I believe this thought? Like I lost at life; I feel like a failure, scum, sad, anxious, angry.

4. How would I feel if I couldn't have the thought? Relieved, free, safe.

5. Turn the thought around to its exact opposite: I am not going to end up like my father.
Any evidence that that's true? Yes, I am with my family, employed, and not addicted to drugs.

———

THOUGHT TO MEDITATE ON:

I am not going to end up like my father.

Example #3

From a widowed mother of 4 children who was chronically stressed and unhappy but not asking for help from her family. She said:

"I should be the strong one."

ANT: "I should be the strong one."

ANT Type(s): Guilt Beating

1. Is it true? Yes.

2. Is it absolutely true with 100 percent certainty? No. At this pace, I am unable to do it all myself.

3. How do I feel when I believe this thought? Defeated, depressed, overwhelmed, like running away.

4. How would I feel if I couldn't have the thought? Like a good mother because I would ask for help and have it when I needed it.

5. Turn the thought around to its exact opposite: I don't have to be the only strong one. I can ask for help.
Any evidence that that's true? Yes, my family has offered, and I can accept their help with gratitude.

_____

THOUGHT TO MEDITATE ON:

I can ask for help.

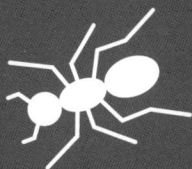

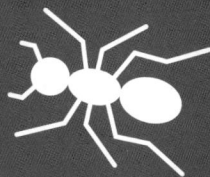

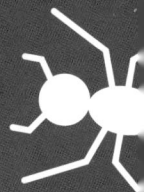

Challenge 100 of Your Worst Thoughts to Change Your Life

One of the first exercises I give patients is to have them write down 100 of their worst ANTs. Then we subject each of them to the elimination process.

If you do this with diligence and thoughtfulness, I promise you will stop fueling emotional distress, end self-defeating thoughts, and be more in control of your happiness and destiny.

The brain learns by repetition. Undisciplined or negative thinking is like a bad habit. The more you engage in it, the more easily the ANTs will attack and take over your mind. These bad thinking habits form through a process called long-term potentiation. When neurons fire together, they wire together, and the negative thoughts become an ingrained part of your life. That is why you need to do this exercise 100 times to teach your brain a new, more rational way of thinking.

Now it's your turn. On the following pages of this booklet, write down 100 of your worst ANTs and then challenge them. You don't have to do this in one sitting. Schedule some time every day to eliminate your worst ANTs.

With practice, you'll become a master ANT killer.

ANT #1: ....

....

ANT TYPE (S): ....

1.   Is it true?

2.   Is it 100% true?

3.   How do you feel when you believe that thought?

4.   Without the thought?

5.   Opposite:

M E D I T A T I O N : ....

....

ANT #2: ....

....

ANT TYPE (S): ....

1.   Is it true?

2.   Is it 100% true?

3.   How do you feel when you believe that thought?

4.   Without the thought?

5.   Opposite:

M E D I T A T I O N : ....

....

ANT #3: ....

....

ANT TYPE (S): ....

1.   Is it true?

2.   Is it 100% true?

3.   How do you feel when you believe that thought?

4.   Without the thought?

5.   Opposite:

MEDITATION: ....

....

ANT #4: ....

....

ANT TYPE (S): ....

1.   Is it true?

2.   Is it 100% true?

3.   How do you feel when you believe that thought?

4.   Without the thought?

5.   Opposite:

MEDITATION: ....

....

ANT #5: ....

....

ANT TYPE (S): ....

1. Is it true?

2. Is it 100% true?

3. How do you feel when you believe that thought?

4. Without the thought?

5. Opposite:

MEDITATION: ....

....

───────────────────────────────

ANT #6: ....

....

ANT TYPE (S): ....

1. Is it true?

2. Is it 100% true?

3. How do you feel when you believe that thought?

4. Without the thought?

5. Opposite:

MEDITATION: ....

....

ANT #7: ....

....

ANT TYPE (S): ....

1.   Is it true?

2.   Is it 100% true?

3.   How do you feel when you believe that thought?

4.   Without the thought?

5.   Opposite:

MEDITATION: ....

....

ANT #8: ....

....

ANT TYPE (S): ....

1.   Is it true?

2.   Is it 100% true?

3.   How do you feel when you believe that thought?

4.   Without the thought?

5.   Opposite:

MEDITATION: ....

....

ANT #9: ....

....

ANT TYPE (S): ....

1.   Is it true?

2.   Is it 100% true?

3.   How do you feel when you believe that thought?

4.   Without the thought?

5.   Opposite:

MEDITATION: ....

....

ANT #10: ....

....

ANT TYPE (S): ....

1.   Is it true?

2.   Is it 100% true?

3.   How do you feel when you believe that thought?

4.   Without the thought?

5.   Opposite:

MEDITATION: ....

....

ANT #11: ....

....

ANT TYPE (S): ....

1.   Is it true?

2.   Is it 100% true?

3.   How do you feel when you believe that thought?

4.   Without the thought?

5.   Opposite:

MEDITATION: ....

....

_____

ANT #12: ....

....

ANT TYPE (S): ....

1.   Is it true?

2.   Is it 100% true?

3.   How do you feel when you believe that thought?

4.   Without the thought?

5.   Opposite:

MEDITATION: ....

....

ANT #13: ....

....

ANT TYPE (S): ....

1.   Is it true?

2.   Is it 100% true?

3.   How do you feel when you believe that thought?

4.   Without the thought?

5.   Opposite:

MEDITATION: ....

....

_____

ANT #14: ....

....

ANT TYPE (S): ....

1.   Is it true?

2.   Is it 100% true?

3.   How do you feel when you believe that thought?

4.   Without the thought?

5.   Opposite:

MEDITATION: ....

....

ANT #15: ....

....

ANT TYPE (S): ....

1.   Is it true?

2.   Is it 100% true?

3.   How do you feel when you believe that thought?

4.   Without the thought?

5.   Opposite:

MEDITATION: ....

....

ANT #16: ....

....

ANT TYPE (S): ....

1.   Is it true?

2.   Is it 100% true?

3.   How do you feel when you believe that thought?

4.   Without the thought?

5.   Opposite:

MEDITATION: ....

....

ANT #17: ....

....

ANT TYPE (S): ....

1.   Is it true?

2.   Is it 100% true?

3.   How do you feel when you believe that thought?

4.   Without the thought?

5.   Opposite:

MEDITATION: ....

....

_____

ANT #18: ....

....

ANT TYPE (S): ....

1.   Is it true?

2.   Is it 100% true?

3.   How do you feel when you believe that thought?

4.   Without the thought?

5.   Opposite:

MEDITATION: ....

....

ANT #19: ....

....

ANT TYPE (S): ....

1.   Is it true?

2.   Is it 100% true?

3.   How do you feel when you believe that thought?

4.   Without the thought?

5.   Opposite:

MEDITATION: ....

....

_____

ANT #20: ....

....

ANT TYPE (S): ....

1.   Is it true?

2.   Is it 100% true?

3.   How do you feel when you believe that thought?

4.   Without the thought?

5.   Opposite:

MEDITATION: ....

....

ANT #21: ....

....

ANT TYPE (S): ....

1.   Is it true?

2.   Is it 100% true?

3.   How do you feel when you believe that thought?

4.   Without the thought?

5.   Opposite:

MEDITATION: ....

....

ANT #22: ....

....

ANT TYPE (S): ....

1.   Is it true?

2.   Is it 100% true?

3.   How do you feel when you believe that thought?

4.   Without the thought?

5.   Opposite:

MEDITATION: ....

....

ANT #23: ....

....

ANT TYPE (S): ....

1.   Is it true?

2.   Is it 100% true?

3.   How do you feel when you believe that thought?

4.   Without the thought?

5.   Opposite:

MEDITATION: ....

....

———————————————————————————————————————

ANT #24: ....

....

ANT TYPE (S): ....

1.   Is it true?

2.   Is it 100% true?

3.   How do you feel when you believe that thought?

4.   Without the thought?

5.   Opposite:

MEDITATION: ....

....

ANT #25: ....

....

ANT TYPE (S): ....

1.   Is it true?

2.   Is it 100% true?

3.   How do you feel when you believe that thought?

4.   Without the thought?

5.   Opposite:

M E D I T A T I O N : ....

....

_____

ANT #26: ....

....

ANT TYPE (S): ....

1.   Is it true?

2.   Is it 100% true?

3.   How do you feel when you believe that thought?

4.   Without the thought?

5.   Opposite:

M E D I T A T I O N : ....

....

ANT #27: ....

....

ANT TYPE (S): ....

1.   Is it true?

2.   Is it 100% true?

3.   How do you feel when you believe that thought?

4.   Without the thought?

5.   Opposite:

MEDITATION: ....

....

_____

ANT #28: ....

....

ANT TYPE (S): ....

1.   Is it true?

2.   Is it 100% true?

3.   How do you feel when you believe that thought?

4.   Without the thought?

5.   Opposite:

MEDITATION: ....

....

ANT #29: ....

....

ANT TYPE (S): ....

1.   Is it true?

2.   Is it 100% true?

3.   How do you feel when you believe that thought?

4.   Without the thought?

5.   Opposite:

MEDITATION: ....

....

_____

ANT #30: ....

....

ANT TYPE (S): ....

1.   Is it true?

2.   Is it 100% true?

3.   How do you feel when you believe that thought?

4.   Without the thought?

5.   Opposite:

MEDITATION: ....

....

ANT #31: ....

....

ANT TYPE (S): ....

1.   Is it true?

2.   Is it 100% true?

3.   How do you feel when you believe that thought?

4.   Without the thought?

5.   Opposite:

MEDITATION: ....

....

ANT #32: ....

....

ANT TYPE (S): ....

1.   Is it true?

2.   Is it 100% true?

3.   How do you feel when you believe that thought?

4.   Without the thought?

5.   Opposite:

MEDITATION: ....

....

ANT #33: ....

....

ANT TYPE (S): ....

1.   Is it true?

2.   Is it 100% true?

3.   How do you feel when you believe that thought?

4.   Without the thought?

5.   Opposite:

MEDITATION: ....

....

ANT #34: ....

....

ANT TYPE (S): ....

1.   Is it true?

2.   Is it 100% true?

3.   How do you feel when you believe that thought?

4.   Without the thought?

5.   Opposite:

MEDITATION: ....

....

ANT #35: ....

....

ANT TYPE (S): ....

1.   Is it true?

2.   Is it 100% true?

3.   How do you feel when you believe that thought?

4.   Without the thought?

5.   Opposite:

MEDITATION: ....

....

_____

ANT #36: ....

....

ANT TYPE (S): ....

1.   Is it true?

2.   Is it 100% true?

3.   How do you feel when you believe that thought?

4.   Without the thought?

5.   Opposite:

MEDITATION: ....

....

ANT #37: ....

....

ANT TYPE (S): ....

1. Is it true?

2. Is it 100% true?

3. How do you feel when you believe that thought?

4. Without the thought?

5. Opposite:

MEDITATION: ....

....

_____

ANT #38: ....

....

ANT TYPE (S): ....

1. Is it true?

2. Is it 100% true?

3. How do you feel when you believe that thought?

4. Without the thought?

5. Opposite:

MEDITATION: ....

....

ANT #39: ....

....

ANT TYPE (S): ....

1.   Is it true?

2.   Is it 100% true?

3.   How do you feel when you believe that thought?

4.   Without the thought?

5.   Opposite:

MEDITATION: ....

....

ANT #40: ....

....

ANT TYPE (S): ....

1.   Is it true?

2.   Is it 100% true?

3.   How do you feel when you believe that thought?

4.   Without the thought?

5.   Opposite:

MEDITATION: ....

....

ANT #41: ....

....

ANT TYPE (S): ....

1.   Is it true?

2.   Is it 100% true?

3.   How do you feel when you believe that thought?

4.   Without the thought?

5.   Opposite:

MEDITATION: ....

....

_____

ANT #42: ....

....

ANT TYPE (S): ....

1.   Is it true?

2.   Is it 100% true?

3.   How do you feel when you believe that thought?

4.   Without the thought?

5.   Opposite:

MEDITATION: ....

....

ANT #43: ....

....

ANT TYPE (S): ....

1.   Is it true?

2.   Is it 100% true?

3.   How do you feel when you believe that thought?

4.   Without the thought?

5.   Opposite:

MEDITATION: ....

....

ANT #44: ....

....

ANT TYPE (S): ....

1.   Is it true?

2.   Is it 100% true?

3.   How do you feel when you believe that thought?

4.   Without the thought?

5.   Opposite:

MEDITATION: ....

....

ANT #45: ....

....

ANT TYPE (S): ....

1.   Is it true?

2.   Is it 100% true?

3.   How do you feel when you believe that thought?

4.   Without the thought?

5.   Opposite:

MEDITATION: ....

....

ANT #46: ....

....

ANT TYPE (S): ....

1.   Is it true?

2.   Is it 100% true?

3.   How do you feel when you believe that thought?

4.   Without the thought?

5.   Opposite:

MEDITATION: ....

....

ANT #47: ....

....

ANT TYPE (S): ....

1.   Is it true?

2.   Is it 100% true?

3.   How do you feel when you believe that thought?

4.   Without the thought?

5.   Opposite:

MEDITATION: ....

....

_____

ANT #48: ....

....

ANT TYPE (S): ....

1.   Is it true?

2.   Is it 100% true?

3.   How do you feel when you believe that thought?

4.   Without the thought?

5.   Opposite:

MEDITATION: ....

....

ANT #49: ....

....

ANT TYPE (S): ....

1.   Is it true?

2.   Is it 100% true?

3.   How do you feel when you believe that thought?

4.   Without the thought?

5.   Opposite:

MEDITATION: ....

....

_____

ANT #50: ....

....

ANT TYPE (S): ....

1.   Is it true?

2.   Is it 100% true?

3.   How do you feel when you believe that thought?

4.   Without the thought?

5.   Opposite:

MEDITATION: ....

....

ANT #51: ....

....

ANT TYPE (S): ....

1.   Is it true?

2.   Is it 100% true?

3.   How do you feel when you believe that thought?

4.   Without the thought?

5.   Opposite:

MEDITATION: ....

....

ANT #52: ....

....

ANT TYPE (S): ....

1.   Is it true?

2.   Is it 100% true?

3.   How do you feel when you believe that thought?

4.   Without the thought?

5.   Opposite:

MEDITATION: ....

....

ANT #53: ....

....

ANT TYPE (S): ....

1.   Is it true?

2.   Is it 100% true?

3.   How do you feel when you believe that thought?

4.   Without the thought?

5.   Opposite:

MEDITATION: ....

....

_____

ANT #54: ....

....

ANT TYPE (S): ....

1.   Is it true?

2.   Is it 100% true?

3.   How do you feel when you believe that thought?

4.   Without the thought?

5.   Opposite:

MEDITATION: ....

....

ANT #55: ....

....

ANT TYPE (S): ....

1.   Is it true?

2.   Is it 100% true?

3.   How do you feel when you believe that thought?

4.   Without the thought?

5.   Opposite:

MEDITATION: ....

....

ANT #56: ....

....

ANT TYPE (S): ....

1.   Is it true?

2.   Is it 100% true?

3.   How do you feel when you believe that thought?

4.   Without the thought?

5.   Opposite:

MEDITATION: ....

....

ANT #57: ....

....

ANT TYPE (S): ....

1.   Is it true?

2.   Is it 100% true?

3.   How do you feel when you believe that thought?

4.   Without the thought?

5.   Opposite:

MEDITATION: ....

....

ANT #58: ....

....

ANT TYPE (S): ....

1.   Is it true?

2.   Is it 100% true?

3.   How do you feel when you believe that thought?

4.   Without the thought?

5.   Opposite:

MEDITATION: ....

....

ANT #59: ....

....

ANT TYPE (S): ....

1.   Is it true?

2.   Is it 100% true?

3.   How do you feel when you believe that thought?

4.   Without the thought?

5.   Opposite:

MEDITATION: ....

....

ANT #60: ....

....

ANT TYPE (S): ....

1.   Is it true?

2.   Is it 100% true?

3.   How do you feel when you believe that thought?

4.   Without the thought?

5.   Opposite:

MEDITATION: ....

....

ANT #61: ....

....

ANT TYPE (S): ....

1.   Is it true?

2.   Is it 100% true?

3.   How do you feel when you believe that thought?

4.   Without the thought?

5.   Opposite:

MEDITATION: ....

....

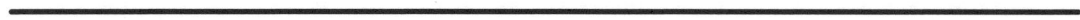

ANT #62: ....

....

ANT TYPE (S): ....

1.   Is it true?

2.   Is it 100% true?

3.   How do you feel when you believe that thought?

4.   Without the thought?

5.   Opposite:

MEDITATION: ....

....

ANT #63: ....

....

ANT TYPE (S): ....

1.   Is it true?

2.   Is it 100% true?

3.   How do you feel when you believe that thought?

4.   Without the thought?

5.   Opposite:

MEDITATION: ....

....

_____

ANT #64: ....

....

ANT TYPE (S): ....

1.   Is it true?

2.   Is it 100% true?

3.   How do you feel when you believe that thought?

4.   Without the thought?

5.   Opposite:

MEDITATION: ....

....

ANT #65: ....

....

ANT TYPE (S): ....

1.   Is it true?

2.   Is it 100% true?

3.   How do you feel when you believe that thought?

4.   Without the thought?

5.   Opposite:

MEDITATION: ....

....

ANT #66: ....

....

ANT TYPE (S): ....

1.   Is it true?

2.   Is it 100% true?

3.   How do you feel when you believe that thought?

4.   Without the thought?

5.   Opposite:

MEDITATION: ....

....

ANT #67: ....

....

ANT TYPE (S): ....

1.   Is it true?

2.   Is it 100% true?

3.   How do you feel when you believe that thought?

4.   Without the thought?

5.   Opposite:

MEDITATION: ....

....

ANT #68: ....

....

ANT TYPE (S): ....

1.   Is it true?

2.   Is it 100% true?

3.   How do you feel when you believe that thought?

4.   Without the thought?

5.   Opposite:

MEDITATION: ....

....

ANT #69: ....

....

ANT TYPE (S): ....

1.   Is it true?

2.   Is it 100% true?

3.   How do you feel when you believe that thought?

4.   Without the thought?

5.   Opposite:

MEDITATION: ....

....

_____

ANT #70: ....

....

ANT TYPE (S): ....

1.   Is it true?

2.   Is it 100% true?

3.   How do you feel when you believe that thought?

4.   Without the thought?

5.   Opposite:

MEDITATION: ....

....

ANT #71: ....

....

ANT TYPE (S): ....

1. Is it true?

2. Is it 100% true?

3. How do you feel when you believe that thought?

4. Without the thought?

5. Opposite:

M E D I T A T I O N : ....

....

ANT #72: ....

....

ANT TYPE (S): ....

1. Is it true?

2. Is it 100% true?

3. How do you feel when you believe that thought?

4. Without the thought?

5. Opposite:

M E D I T A T I O N : ....

....

ANT #73: ....

....

ANT TYPE (S): ....

1.   Is it true?

2.   Is it 100% true?

3.   How do you feel when you believe that thought?

4.   Without the thought?

5.   Opposite:

MEDITATION: ....

....

ANT #74: ....

....

ANT TYPE (S): ....

1.   Is it true?

2.   Is it 100% true?

3.   How do you feel when you believe that thought?

4.   Without the thought?

5.   Opposite:

MEDITATION: ....

....

ANT #75: ....

....

ANT TYPE (S): ....

1.   Is it true?

2.   Is it 100% true?

3.   How do you feel when you believe that thought?

4.   Without the thought?

5.   Opposite:

MEDITATION: ....

....

_____

ANT #76: ....

....

ANT TYPE (S): ....

1.   Is it true?

2.   Is it 100% true?

3.   How do you feel when you believe that thought?

4.   Without the thought?

5.   Opposite:

MEDITATION: ....

....

ANT #77: ....

....

ANT TYPE (S): ....

1. Is it true?

2. Is it 100% true?

3. How do you feel when you believe that thought?

4. Without the thought?

5. Opposite:

MEDITATION: ....

....

ANT #78: ....

....

ANT TYPE (S): ....

1. Is it true?

2. Is it 100% true?

3. How do you feel when you believe that thought?

4. Without the thought?

5. Opposite:

MEDITATION: ....

....

ANT #79: ....

....

ANT TYPE (S): ....

1.   Is it true?

2.   Is it 100% true?

3.   How do you feel when you believe that thought?

4.   Without the thought?

5.   Opposite:

MEDITATION: ....

....

ANT #80: ....

....

ANT TYPE (S): ....

1.   Is it true?

2.   Is it 100% true?

3.   How do you feel when you believe that thought?

4.   Without the thought?

5.   Opposite:

MEDITATION: ....

....

ANT #81: ....

....

ANT TYPE (S): ....

1.   Is it true?

2.   Is it 100% true?

3.   How do you feel when you believe that thought?

4.   Without the thought?

5.   Opposite:

MEDITATION: ....

....

———————————————————————————————————

ANT #82: ....

....

ANT TYPE (S): ....

1.   Is it true?

2.   Is it 100% true?

3.   How do you feel when you believe that thought?

4.   Without the thought?

5.   Opposite:

MEDITATION: ....

....

ANT #83:..

....

ANT TYPE (S): ....

1.   Is it true?

2.   Is it 100% true?

3.   How do you feel when you believe that thought?

4.   Without the thought?

5.   Opposite:

MEDITATION: ....

....

_____

ANT #84: ....

....

ANT TYPE (S): ....

1.   Is it true?

2.   Is it 100% true?

3.   How do you feel when you believe that thought?

4.   Without the thought?

5.   Opposite:

MEDITATION: ....

....

ANT #85: ....

....

ANT TYPE (S): ....

1. Is it true?

2. Is it 100% true?

3. How do you feel when you believe that thought?

4. Without the thought?

5. Opposite:

MEDITATION: ....

....

ANT #86: ....

....

ANT TYPE (S): ....

1. Is it true?

2. Is it 100% true?

3. How do you feel when you believe that thought?

4. Without the thought?

5. Opposite:

MEDITATION: ....

....

ANT #87: ....

....

ANT TYPE (S): ....

1.   Is it true?

2.   Is it 100% true?

3.   How do you feel when you believe that thought?

4.   Without the thought?

5.   Opposite:

MEDITATION: ....

....

ANT #88: ....

....

ANT TYPE (S): ....

1.   Is it true?

2.   Is it 100% true?

3.   How do you feel when you believe that thought?

4.   Without the thought?

5.   Opposite:

MEDITATION: ....

....

ANT #89: ....

....

ANT TYPE (S): ....

1.   Is it true?

2.   Is it 100% true?

3.   How do you feel when you believe that thought?

4.   Without the thought?

5.   Opposite:

MEDITATION: ....

....

ANT #90: ....

....

ANT TYPE (S): ....

1.   Is it true?

2.   Is it 100% true?

3.   How do you feel when you believe that thought?

4.   Without the thought?

5.   Opposite:

MEDITATION: ....

....

ANT #91: ....

....

ANT TYPE (S): ....

1. Is it true?

2. Is it 100% true?

3. How do you feel when you believe that thought?

4. Without the thought?

5. Opposite:

MEDITATION: ....

....

_____

ANT #92: ....

....

ANT TYPE (S): ....

1. Is it true?

2. Is it 100% true?

3. How do you feel when you believe that thought?

4. Without the thought?

5. Opposite:

MEDITATION: ....

....

ANT #93: ....

....

ANT TYPE (S): ....

1.   Is it true?

2.   Is it 100% true?

3.   How do you feel when you believe that thought?

4.   Without the thought?

5.   Opposite:

MEDITATION: ....

....

ANT #94: ....

....

ANT TYPE (S): ....

1.   Is it true?

2.   Is it 100% true?

3.   How do you feel when you believe that thought?

4.   Without the thought?

5.   Opposite:

MEDITATION: ....

....

ANT #95: ....

....

ANT TYPE (S): ....

1.   Is it true?

2.   Is it 100% true?

3.   How do you feel when you believe that thought?

4.   Without the thought?

5.   Opposite:

MEDITATION: ....

....

ANT #96: ....

....

ANT TYPE (S): ....

1.   Is it true?

2.   Is it 100% true?

3.   How do you feel when you believe that thought?

4.   Without the thought?

5.   Opposite:

MEDITATION: ....

....

ANT #97: ....

....

ANT TYPE (S): ....

1.   Is it true?

2.   Is it 100% true?

3.   How do you feel when you believe that thought?

4.   Without the thought?

5.   Opposite:

MEDITATION: ....

....

ANT #98: ....

....

ANT TYPE (S): ....

1.   Is it true?

2.   Is it 100% true?

3.   How do you feel when you believe that thought?

4.   Without the thought?

5.   Opposite:

MEDITATION: ....

....

ANT #99:..
....

ANT TYPE (S): ....

1.   Is it true?

2.   Is it 100% true?

3.   How do you feel when you believe that thought?

4.   Without the thought?

5.   Opposite:

MEDITATION: ....
....

ANT #100: ....
....

ANT TYPE (S): ....

1.   Is it true?

2.   Is it 100% true?

3.   How do you feel when you believe that thought?

4.   Without the thought?

5.   Opposite:

MEDITATION: ....
....

THE NEXT STEP:

Make ANT-Killing a Daily Habit

Congratulations!

You have completed one of the most powerful tools to end negative thinking patterns, improve your moods, and decrease anxiety. But this isn't the end. Killing the ANTs takes practice. You can't just do this exercise once and think you've mastered your thinking patterns.

You need to make ANT killing a daily practice.

When you make it an everyday routine, you will feel freer, less anxious and depressed, and less trapped in past hurts or losses.